Energize Your Essence

A Comprehensive Recovery Blueprint"

Meta J. Myers

Copyright

Disclaimer:

The material introduced in "Energize Your Essence:A Comprehensive Recovery Blueprint"by Meta J. Myers is planned for general enlightening purposes as it were. Meta J. Myers isn't responsible for any mix-ups or exclusions and repudiates any liability regarding the results acquired from the utilization of this data. The data is definitely not a substitute for proficient counsel, conclusion, or treatment.

It is recommended that readers seek specialized, individualized assistance. Meta J. Myers disclaims all responsibility for decisions made or actions taken based on the information provided, as well as liability for any damages or losses resulting from the use of this publication, either directly or indirectly. By getting to and utilizing this distribution, you consent to the circumstances referenced in this disclaimer.

About the author

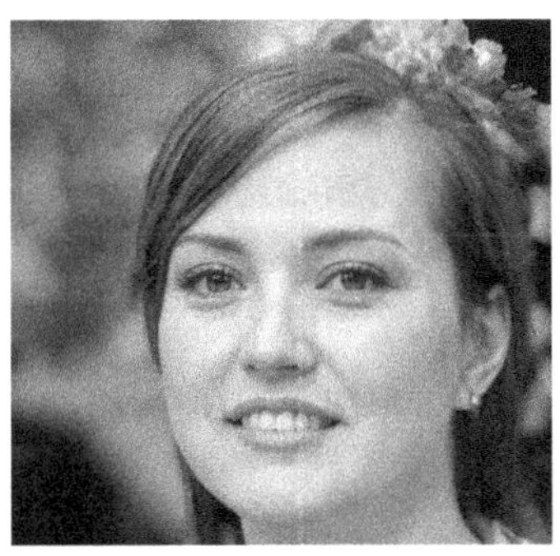

Meta J. Myers, the insightful author behind "Energize Your Essence: A Comprehensive Recovery Blueprint," is a passionate supporter for overall well-being. With a foundation in brain science and a profound obligation to engaging individuals, Meta carries an abundance of information to the universe of self-improvement.

Known for her drawing recorded as a hard copy style and delicate methodology, Meta mixes her scholastic information with genuine bits of knowledge to direct pursuers on an extraordinary excursion toward rejuvenating their pith.. Her commitment to the study of energy dynamics, resilience-building, and mindful living is obvious in the pages of this comprehensive blueprint.

Meta is not just an author but a health enthusiast dedicated to helping people manage the complexities of modern life. Drawing inspiration from her own experiences and studies, she aims to inspire others to reclaim control over their energy and create a life filled with continued vigor and purpose.

Table of contents

INTRODUCTION..**10**

   UNDERSTANDING THE ESSENCE OF ENERGY 12

   RECOGNIZING THE SIGNS OF DEPLETION.......17

CHAPTER 1:THE POWER OF AWARENESS............ 22

   CULTIVATING SELF-AWARENESS......................26

   IDENTIFYING ENERGY DRAINS.......................... 31

CHAPTER 2: BUILDING RESILIENCE......................36

   STRENGTHENING MENTAL RESILIENCE...........40

   EMOTIONAL RESILIENCE.................................. 46

CHAPTER 3: MINDFUL REJUVENATION..................52

   EXPLORING MINDFULNESS PRACTICES.......... 56

   INTEGRATING MINDFUL HABITS INTO DAILY
   LIFE... 62

**CHAPTER 4: REVITALIZING YOUR PHYSICAL CORE
67**

   PRIORITIZING SLEEP AND RESTORATION........73

   NOURISHING YOUR BODY FOR OPTIMAL
   ENERGY...77

CHAPTER 5: CONNECTING WITH PURPOSE..........84

   REDISCOVERING YOUR PASSION..................... 89

   ALIGNING YOUR ACTIVITIES WITH YOUR

VALUES..94

CHAPTER 6: SOCIAL ENERGIZERS.......................100

   BUILDING SUPPORTIVE CONNECTIONS.........105

   SETTING BOUNDARIES FOR HEALTHY RELATIONSHIPS..111

CHAPTER 7: ENERGIZING WORK AND PRODUCTIVITY..115

   BALANCING WORKLOAD AND PERSONAL TIME.. 119

   ENHANCING PRODUCTIVITY THROUGH ENERGY MANAGEMENT....................................124

CHAPTER 8: CREATIVITY AND PLAY......................130

   TAPPING INTO CREATIVE ENERGIES.............135

   EMBRACING PLAY AND LEISURE....................139

CHAPTER 9: OVERCOMING OBSTACLES.............144

   IDENTIFYING AND OVERCOMING BARRIERS TO RECOVERY..148

   LEARNING FROM SETBACKS...........................154

CONCLUSION..160

INTRODUCTION

Welcome to "Energize Your Essence: A Comprehensive Recovery Blueprint". In the rushing of our day to day routines, keeping a feeling of energy and equilibrium can frequently feel like a tricky objective. This guide is designed as a road map for navigating the challenges of modern life and provides a comprehensive strategy for reviving your energy and reclaiming tranquility.

In the following chapters, we dig into the core of energy—exploring the intricate interplay of physical well-being, mental resilience, and thoughtful living. Each part is meant to empower you with practical insights and actionable strategies, leading you towards a renewed sense of purpose, connection, and excitement.

As we start on this journey together, remember that the way to recovery is unique for each person. Whether you seek to overcome fatigue, alleviate worry, or simply improve your general well-being, "Energize Your Essence" is here to inspire and support your personal change.

Let the journey begin as we discover the keys to unlocking your full potential and revitalizing your soul.

UNDERSTANDING THE ESSENCE OF ENERGY

Energy has a significant role in the realm of human experience. It is the same thing that gives us life and vitality and drives our emotions, ideas, and behaviors. To truly reclaim our identity, we must first embark on a journey of self-discovery and comprehend the intricate connections between our physical, mental, and emotional well-being.This entails appreciating restful sleep, exercising frequently, and providing our bodies with healthy meals.

Building a healthy mind, filling our minds with affirmations, and engaging in mindfulness exercises are all crucial for promoting inner calm and tranquility. This involves valuing peaceful rest, practicing much of the time, and giving our bodies good feasts.

Building a sound psyche, filling our brains with confirmations, and participating in care practices are pivotal for advancing inward quiet and serenity. A vital component of emotional health is receiving compassion and gratitude for both ourselves and other people.

These components work together to produce a dynamic equilibrium in our lives—a harmonious balance that makes it possible for our energy to flow freely. This is what true vitality is all about—a feeling of being strong, connected, and fully alive.

Crucial Advice for Revitalizing Your Essence

•**Nourish Your Body:** Give your body nutrient-dense meals to keep it full throughout the day. Steer clear of sugary drinks, processed meals, and excessive coffee.

•**Embrace Regular Development:** Participate in proactive tasks that you like, like riding, moving, swimming, or fast strolling. On most days of the week, attempt to get in something like 30 minutes of moderate-power exercise.

To give your body the time it needs to unwind and recover, make getting 7-8 hours of quality sleep a priority each night. Establish a calming routine at night and a regular sleep schedule.

•**Foster Care:** Try mindfulness exercises like deep breathing or meditation to unwind, reduce stress, and sharpen your attention.

•**Practice appreciation**: Offer thanks consistently for the great parts of your life to encourage prosperity and regard.

•**Foster social networks**: Assemble a supportive network of people that encourage and elevate you.

Follow Your Interests: Invest time in things that make you happy and meaningful so that your true passions can pique your curiosity.

Recall that awakening your soul is a journey, not a destination. Accept the journey of self-discovery, take care of your body, mind, and emotions, and see as your energy levels rise to a life full of vitality, purpose, and genuine connection.

RECOGNIZING THE SIGNS OF DEPLETION

Have you ever felt more like a faltering candle than a roaring bonfire? Everybody has experienced depletion—those moments when they feel low on spirit, lose their enthusiasm for life, and feel short on energy. But the secret to regaining your glow is knowing the warning signals.

Let's examine a few typical depletion signals:

Physical:

• Fatigue: Constantly feeling exhausted, even after getting enough rest.

•Aches and pains: Muscle strain, headaches, or unexplained physical discomfort.

•Ankle pain, insomnia, or changes in appetite or sleep: eating too much or too little.

• Weakened immune system: recurring infections, gastrointestinal issues, or colds.

Emotional:

•Irritability or apathy: Having an easily irritated or uninterested mood.

•Loss of passion or joy: Things that formerly made you feel good now seem mediocre.

• Having trouble concentrating or making decisions: experiencing mental fog or disarray.

•A greater sense of seclusion or withdrawal: avoiding people or activities you formerly enjoyed.

Mental:

• Self-doubt or negative thinking: a persistent inner critic or a fixation on previous transgressions.

•Exhaustion or stress: Difficulty completing obligations or everyday duties.

• Lack of creativity or imagination: Sensing trapped and unable to come up with fresh concepts.

• Cynicism or hopelessness: Perceiving that there is no point in living or that circumstances will never improve.

Recall that depletion is a warning rather than a sanction. It's a reminder to take it easy, relax, and rediscover your passion. You may take action to support your health, mind, and spirit by identifying these indications.

CHAPTER 1: THE POWER OF AWARENESS

Imagine turning a switch and lighting a dark room. That's the power of awareness in "Energize Your Essence." It's the key to turning on your inner light and removing the dark of depletion.

Think of awareness as a spotlight. It shines on the corners of your life, showing what's taking your energy and what sparks your joy.

It helps you see:

1.The energy vampires: Toxic relationships, negative self-talk, and excessive responsibilities that zap your spirit.

2.The secret gems: Activities that make your heart sing, interests that ignite your soul, and times of quiet peace that replenish your well-being.

By developing awareness, you become the master of your energy. You can:

1.Choose wisely: Say "no" to energy drains and favor activities that fill your cup.

2.Nurture your needs: Listen to your body's words and react with rest, movement, or nourishing food.

3.Celebrate small wins: Recognize and respect even the smallest steps towards your goals.

4.Embrace forgiveness: Let go of past hurts and self-blame, freeing up room for joy and growth.

Awareness is a gift, a tool for change. It helps you to step off the hamster wheel of depletion and onto the road of vibrant life. In the next part of "Energize Your Essence," we'll explore practical tasks to develop awareness and spark your inner power. Remember, the light is always within you; awareness is just the dimming switch. Let's turn it up together!

CULTIVATING SELF-AWARENESS

Consider caring for a garden. You must understand what the flowers require in terms of soil, sunshine, and water in order to help them flourish. Being self-aware is similar to taking care of your spiritual garden. Understanding who you are, what you desire, and what drives your personal development is key.

Here are a few simple techniques to cultivate self-awareness and see your soul emerge:

1.Whispers of the Body:

• **Arrival**: Every day, take a minute to reflect. Observe your stance, breathing, and any torments or pressure. Focus on everything your body is saying to you. Does it need to move, relax, or have a healthy meal?

• **Move and groove:** Whether it's dancing, taking a stroll in the outdoors, or stretching, discover what makes your body sing. Forging a connection with your physical self and letting go of stored energy, movement is a powerful technique.

2.Conscientious Eating:

• **Pay attention to your hunger**: Before reaching for a snack, consider if you're actually hungry or whether you're just worn out, anxious, or in need of comfort. Observe how various factors impact your mood and energy levels.

• **Savor the bites:** Eat mindfully and slowly. Take note of the tastes, scents, and textures. Eating mindfully nourishes not only your physical body but also your awareness of your desires and objectives.

3.Echolocation with emotion:

• **Recognize your triggers**: Take note of the things or people that usually sap your energy or cause you to feel bad. It gives you the ability to manage difficult situations and establish reasonable boundaries.

•**Recognize your blessings**: Think about the things that make you smile, laugh, or feel genuinely alive. Cherish those moments and make an effort to do happy things more frequently. It's crucial to visit your happy spots to replenish your soul's energy.

Concise Taming:

•**Catch the reviewer:** Pay attention to your inner critic's critical remarks as they arise. Without passing judgment, acknowledge its presence and then gradually shift your focus to something positive or neutral.

•**Cultivate thankfulness:** Make time every day to acknowledge and appreciate all of life's blessings, no matter how tiny. A lighter, more energetic heart is a joyful heart.

Recall that developing self-awareness is a journey, not a destination. Enjoy the journey of discovering your bright inner soul, be kind to yourself, and acknowledge your progress. In the upcoming section of "Energize Your Essence," we'll discuss how to apply this expanded understanding to make decisions that feed your body, mind, and spirit, resulting in a life full of vitality and happiness.

IDENTIFYING ENERGY DRAINS

Consider yourself a brilliant lamp overflowing with light. Imagine small fractures allowing light to leak out, leaving you feeling dull and empty. Those fissures are your energy drains, the villains robbing you of your enthusiasm for life. But don't worry, they're easier to repair than you think!

Let's take a look at some of the most prevalent energy drains:

People:

•**Nancy the Negative**: Constantly whining, depleting your optimism with dread and gloom.

•**The Energy Vampire**: Constantly drains your energy with negativity or neediness.

•The time band demands your attention without regard for your limits.

Activities:

•**Endless scrolling**: social media rabbit holes that engulf you and leave you feeling depleted.

•Busywork is defined as repetitive duties that drain your motivation.

•**To-Do Overload**: An overloaded plate that stresses and overwhelms you.

Habits:

•Sleep robbers include late-night phone scrolling and coffee excesses that interrupt sleep.
•Sugar crashes, processed foods, and missing meals all contribute to sluggishness.

•**Negative Self-Talk:** The inner critic is always knocking you down and depriving you of your confidence.

Remember, the first step to regaining your strength is to identify your energy drains. Once you've identified the perpetrators, you can take the following steps:

•**Set boundaries:** avoid negative individuals, say no to time wasters, and unsubscribe from energy-sucking social media.

Choose things that stimulate you, delegate or eliminate busywork, and arrange leisure for activities you genuinely like.

Sleeping first, eating well, and taking care of yourself will boost your mental and physical energy.

Negative thoughts ought to be tested. Supplant self-analysis with positive assertions, and focus on your most desirable characteristics.

Empowering yourself to recognize and eliminate energy depletion is analogous to fixing leaks in your light. Soon, you'll be shining brighter than ever, spreading your brilliant spirit to the world. In the next installment of "Energize Your Essence," we'll look at techniques to recharge and refill your energy so that your inner light may shine brightly!

CHAPTER 2: BUILDING RESILIENCE

Consider your essence to be a beautiful castle, colorful, and alive. But, like any fortress, it needs sturdy walls to resist the trials of life. That's where resilience comes in—the mortar that keeps your inner world afloat even as the skies darken.

Here are a few easy strategies to strengthen your resilience and keep your essence energized:

Accept the bounce:

• Regard setbacks as stepping stones: Rather than becoming disheartened by difficulties, regard them as chances to learn and progress. Each reversal strengthens your fortress defenses.

• Center around progress instead of flawlessness: rather than worrying about mistakes, celebrate small accomplishments. Recall that even the mightiest oak started as a little oak seed.

Keep an Eye on Your Moat:

• Nurture your support system: Surround yourself with positive individuals who inspire and boost you up. Your moat is a safe refuge of strength and comfort.

• Exercise self-care: Schedule time for things that fill your cup, like reading, going for a walk, or spending time in nature. Make your health a priority in order to keep your defenses robust.

Sharpen your blades.

• Learn solid procedures to deal with pressure and pessimistic feelings, like contemplation, journaling, or conversing with a specialist. Having devices in your stockpile is fundamental for flexibility.

• Believe in yourself: Develop a positive attitude and self-confidence. You can confront any problem if you trust in your own power.

Remember that developing resilience is a process, not a destination. There may be challenges along the path, but each one will build your inner castle. Keep your resilience muscles flexed, learn from your disappointments, and celebrate your successes. In the following portion of "Energize your essence," we'll take a gander at how to utilize gratefulness and idealism to keep your inward fire bursting hot regardless of what life tosses at you.

STRENGTHENING MENTAL RESILIENCE

Think of your essence as a brilliant flame that is bursting with joy and vitality. But just like any other fire, it needs protection from the rain and wind. That is where mental durability comes in: it goes about as a subtle safeguard to keep your inward fire bursting splendidly even notwithstanding difficulties that could somehow smother it.

Being intellectually strong requires being adaptable as opposed to invulnerable. It is the ability to endure life's storms, bounce back from failures, and carry on with your flame burning brightly. So, how do we build this vital barrier?

The following are some easy actions you can do:

1. Increase Your Self-Awareness

• **Be aware of your triggers:** What circumstances or individuals channel your energy or prompt you to feel awful? Recognizing your weaknesses is the initial step to further developing them.

· **Honor your inborn gifts or capacities**: Which natural capacities or abilities do you have? Acknowledging your advantages gives you more self-assurance and enables you to face challenges head-on.

2. Adopt a Positive Outlook:

•**View issues as opportunities:** Rather of being terrified of failures, view them as opportunities to grow and learn. Keep in mind that every compelling story includes unexpected turns.

• **Practice gratefulness**: No matter how big or small, pay attention to the amazing things in your life. A heart that is grateful finds strength in any circumstance.

3. Invest in your personal development:

•Put away opportunities for exercises that revive your body and brain, such actual work, time spent in nature, or creative pursuits. A tough self is one who is very much refreshed and very much took care of.

•Build strong bonds: Be in the company of kind people who will support and uplift you. Your loved ones can be your compass in choppy waters.

4. Create Well-Being Coping Strategies:

• **Learn how to reduce stress:** Yoga, contemplation, profound breathing, and time spent in nature may all assist you with managing pressure and gloomy feelings in a solid manner.

•**Look for proficient assistance when required**: Try not to be terrified to reach out to a specialist or instructor on the off chance that you're having issues.Consulting with an expert might offer you practical strategies for handling difficult circumstances.

Recall that building mental toughness is a journey, not a destination. There will be highs and lows, but as you overcome each challenge, the light within you will continue to shine. Remember these simple steps, appreciate your victories, and accept the process. You're capable of it!

If you have a vivid essence and a strong mental barrier, you can weather any storm and keep your inner fire shining brightly!

EMOTIONAL RESILIENCE

Consider your essence to be a lovely landscape brimming with vitality and color. However, it, like any garden, needs strong roots to withstand storms and nourish its flowers. That is where close to home flexibility comes in - the profound root foundation that roots your heart and keeps it sound and blooming even despite close to home storms.

Profound strength doesn't suggest being unfeeling; rather, it involves understanding and directing your feelings without permitting them to lead you.It's similar to learning to dance in the rain, transforming a potential storm into an elegant display of inner power. So, how can we nurture this priceless skill?

Here are few easy steps:

1. Understand Your Garden:

•Determine your emotions: Pay attention to your emotions and learn to identify them. Are you worried, annoyed, upset, or happy? Understanding your emotional environment empowers you to control it.

•Accept your emotions: Don't berate yourself for feeling the way you do. Every feeling is genuine and has a purpose. Allow yourself to feel without feeling guilty or ashamed.

2. Feed Your Roots:

•Focus on exercises that renew your close to home prosperity, like investing energy in nature, paying attention to loosening up music, or enjoying leisure activities you like. A heart that has been fostered is a heart that is resilient.

• Establish solid bonds: Encircle yourself with individuals who embrace and figure you out. Realizing you have a protected spot to communicate your sentiments unafraid of being judged is fundamental for profound flexibility.

3. Get ready for Tempests:

•Foster great survival techniques: Learn sound ways of communicating and control your feelings, like composition, conversing with a companion, or working out. Finding positive outlets for your emotions guards your inner garden against emotional damage.

•View setbacks and problems as opportunities for growth: View setbacks and difficulties as opportunities to learn, adapt, and improve your emotional muscles. Remember that even the most beautiful gardens have had to endure storms in order to bloom fully.

4. Commemorate the Sun:

•Exercise gratitude: Concentrate on the wonderful things in your life, no matter how large or tiny. Even in the face of difficulties, a thankful heart finds delight, keeping your garden bright and full of hope.

•Believe in yourself: Remind yourself of your resilience and strength. You've conquered adversity before, and you can do so again. Have faith in your capacity to withstand any emotional storm.

Recall that creating profound flexibility is a cycle, not an objective. There will be events when your nursery is exposed to areas of strength and weighty downpour. However, with careful attention and four easy actions, you can grow a heart that blossoms with bright vigor and elegance, no matter what life throws at you. So, accept the process, celebrate your progress, and watch your essence blossom with the strength of a strong heart.

CHAPTER 3: MINDFUL REJUVENATION

Are you exhausted? Is your radiance fading? You're not by yourself. We are all victims of the burnout cycle, speeding through life on an empty stomach. However, there is a hidden weapon against depletion: conscious renewal.

Consider it a spa for your soul, a chance to rejuvenate your mind, body, and spirit from inside. There are no fad diets or strenuous exercises involved, only easy methods to regain your vivid soul.

Here's your mindful rejuvenation recipe:

• **Move with joy:** Instead of going to the gym, look for things that make you happy. Take a conscious nature stroll, dance in your kitchen, or stretch in the sun. Pay attention to your body and exercise in ways that feel pleasant.

• **Feed wisely**: Forget about restricted diets. Fill your plate with hole, flavorful items that will give you energy. Get rid of the guilt and start listening to your body's hunger signals.

• **Recharge and rest:** Sleep is your superpower. Make it a priority! Make a loosening-up rest custom to help you loosen up and relinquish the burdens of the day. Awaken feeling renewed and prepared for the day.

• **Quiet your psyche**: endure five minutes pondering, doing breathwork, or going for a calm walk in nature. These simple procedures can assist you with quieting your brain and lessening pressure, leaving you feeling focused and peaceful.

•**Express yourself**: Let your inner artist loose! Draw, paint, sing, dance, or simply doodle. Allow your imagination to flow and exhibit your own identity.

• **Share and connect**: Spend time with individuals who inspire and encourage you. Share your experience, join a support group, or simply talk about it. A strong source of energy is connection.

Remember that mindful rejuvenation is a journey rather than a destination. Be patient, enjoy the process of regaining your inner spark, and celebrate your accomplishments. This is your unique route to a life filled with brilliant energy!

EXPLORING MINDFULNESS PRACTICES

Life might feel like an endless to-do list, a swirl of ideas and demands. But what if you could tap into an inner source of energy, a lively core that hums with joy and presence? That's when mindfulness comes in—a hidden ability just waiting to be discovered!

Imagine:

Stress fades away, to be replaced with quiet assurance.

Worries dissipate like mist, to be replaced with a clear, concentrated mind.

Your body vibrates with energy, like a newly charged battery.

Care isn't some enchanted rubbish; it's tied in with concentrating completely on the ongoing second. It resembles shining an electric lamp on your life, highlighting the great and directing you through the terrible with beauty.

So, how can you tap into this enchantment?

To get you started, here are a few easy practices:

1. Inhale Like a Boss:

Your breath is your connection to the current moment. Take a few deep, thoughtful breaths whenever tension strikes. Feel the rise and fall of your stomach, the chilly air in your nostrils, and the warmth out. It resembles squeezing the reset button for your brain and body.

2. Body Scan: Get to Know Your Form:

Close your eyes, and mentally go through your body. Feel the earth beneath your toes by wriggling them. Pay attention to how you feel in your head, chest, and limbs as you get up. This isn't tied in with assessing your body; rather, it is tied in with embracing it as your astonishing life-emotionally supportive network.

3. Nature Fix: Green Recharge:

Step outside and permit nature to do its thing. Feel the sun all over, the breeze in your hair, and the ground underneath your feet. Take in the hints of larks, the stirring of leaves, and the murmuring of a stream. Nature joins you to an option that could be more significant than yourself, mixing you with essentialness and harmony.

4. Gratitude Groove: Find Joy Within:

Every day, take a moment to appreciate the little things. A hot cup of coffee, a child's giggle, and a fiery sunset. Gratitude turns your emphasis from what is lacking to what is abundant, increasing your delight.

Remember:

Mindfulness is a journey, not an end point. Be kind to yourself, rejoice in minor achievements, and have fun! These are a couple of ideas to kick you off. Experiment, discover what works for you, and build your own particular arsenal for inner transformation.

With a little mindfulness magic, you'll notice your essence radiating with renewed vigor, ready to take on anything life throws at you!

Make it a habit to practice mindfulness! Incorporate it into regular activities such as walking, eating, and even conversing. Every moment is an opportunity to reconnect with your current self and access your inner strength.

So, go forth and discover the wonders of mindfulness! Remember that you've got this, and your essence is just waiting to be activated!

INTEGRATING MINDFUL HABITS INTO DAILY LIFE

Life is a whirlwind of work, errands, and, at times, complete chaos. But what if you could add a hidden ingredient - mindfulness magic - to convert that smoothie into a powerhouse? Please, yes!

1.Mindfulness isn't some expensive retreat; it's about focusing your attention completely on the current moment, as if you were squeezing the most juicy pieces out of life. What's more, the finest part? You may easily incorporate it into your everyday routine:

2.Morning Brew: Start your day with a 5-minute breath meditation. Sit motionless, eyes closed, and concentrate on your breathing. Feel it fill your lungs and then softly expel it. Voila! A peaceful, centering start to your day.

3.Café Break Don't gulp, Bliss! Enjoy your coffee slowly. Take note of the perfume, the warmth in your palms, and the flavor that dances on your tongue. Each sip becomes a mini-moment of happiness.

3.Workday Zen: Put an end to multitasking! When working on a task, give it your undivided attention. Put your phone aside, shut any superfluous tabs, and concentrate on your current task. You'll finish tasks faster and feel less stressed.

4.Lunchtime Escape: Take a mindful stroll instead of working at your desk. Take in everything you see, hear, and smell around you. Feel the sun everywhere and the breeze in your hair. Connecting with nature can help you refuel.

5.Dinner Dance: Make meals a conscious feast rather than a fuel-up. Slowly chew, relish each bite, and enjoy the company (even if it's just you!). Make supper an opportunity to nurture both your body and your spirit.

6.Tech Timeout: Before going to bed, turn off all screens and take a thoughtful tech break. Spend 10 minutes alone with yourself, stretching, reading a book, or simply sitting in solitude and observing your thoughts. Unplug your device to replenish your internal battery.

7.Keep in mind that consistency is essential! Sprinkle these thoughtful behaviors throughout your day like rays of sunlight. Be kind to yourself, don't pass judgment, and have fun!

8.Bonus Tip: Spread the mindfulness love! Inviting friends and family to join you on mindful walks, lunches, or coffee breaks is a good idea. You may produce a calming and joyful ripple effect by working together.

So go ahead and sprinkle! Watch your essence glow with vitality, fuelled by the delectableness of attentive living. You can do it!

CHAPTER 4: REVITALIZING YOUR PHYSICAL CORE

Deep within you is a hidden power source, a reservoir of physical vigor just waiting to be discovered. It's not a mythological dragon's treasure, but your own core, the muscle powerhouse that supports your posture, mobility, and general well-being. Unleashing its power may change your life by infusing it with the vivid buzz of physical strength and presence.

Here's how to transform your core into a positive energy generator:

1. Activate the Powerhouse:

Begin small! Avoid crunches in favor of more moderate movements such as planks or bird-dogs. Feel your core muscles contract, supporting and balancing your body. Hold for a few breaths, then exhale while enjoying the slight burn. It's not about getting a six-pack, but rather about connecting with your body's inherent strength.

2. Deep Breathing:

Keep in mind that your core and your breath are great friends. Deep, deliberate breaths engage your diaphragm, which is directly connected to your core muscles. With each inhale, feel your belly expand, bringing strength into your center. Exhale completely, releasing all tension and stress. Every breath is a mini-workout for your core, recharging you from inside.

3. Move with Purpose:

Forget the treadmill at the gym! Convert regular activities into core-strengthening exercises. Engage your core mindfully whether washing the chores, gardening, or even walking the dog. As you bend, twist, and reach, notice the tiny engagement. Small motions performed with mindfulness can have a significant impact.

4. Pay Attention to Your Body:

Maintain your limits! Do not push yourself through pain or suffering. Adjust or take a break if something feels odd. Listen to your body's whispers and heed its requirements since it is your smart guide. Remember that the slogan of a happy core is growth, not perfection.

5. Appreciate the Journey:

Your ultimate source of energy is joy! Find methods to exercise that make you laugh and smile. Dance to your favorite music, try a silly yoga stance, or simply wiggle to the beat of life. Let go of expectations and enjoy the freedom that comes from moving your body in ways that feel pleasant.

Remember:

Revitalizing your physical core is about more than simply getting chiseled abs; it's about gaining a greater sense of power and confidence. You'll move more fluidly, exude vigor, and feel more at home in your own skin. Tune in to your core, pay attention to its whispers, and see your essence shine with renewed vigor!

Bonus Tip: Spread the love! Inviting friends and family to join you for mindful walks, movement breaks, or even goofy dance parties is a great way to start the day. You may generate a ripple effect of physical and emotional well-being by working together.

Go forth and discover your inner strength! You'll learn the actual meaning of "energize your essence" from the ground up with a little awareness and delight.

PRIORITIZING SLEEP AND RESTORATION

We've all felt the sluggishness and exhaustion that resulted from not getting sufficient rest. Then again, focusing on rest and reclamation implies something beyond staying away from weakness; it likewise implies releasing the brilliant capability of your embodiment.Think of it as a kind of internal battery recharge that will leave you energized, laser-focused, and prepared to shine!

1. Sleeping is the Best Recharge

•Aim for 7-8 hours each night of restful sleep. Depending on your unique needs, this could change somewhat, but most adults do well in this range.

• Create a routine at night that tells your body when it's time to unwind. Peruse a book, wash up, or partake in a loosening up music to assist you with loosening up. Give yourself essentially an hour prior to bed to try not to utilize screens.

•Decorate your sleeping space as a haven. Invest on soft bedding, a comfortable mattress, and blackout curtains if needed. Keep the temperature down and the noise level down.

2. Healing Ceremonies Outside of Sleep:

•Be in the present: Throughout the day, take regular breaks to disconnect from technology and focus on being in the now. Stretch, go on a walk, or simply sit quietly and observe your surroundings.

• Support your body: To give your body the assets it requires to mend and recover, eat an eating routine wealthy in natural products, vegetables, and entire grains. Remember to remain hydrated!

• Move your body: Getting more exercise is a great way to reduce stress and boost energy. However, remember that light movement is crucial. Pick pastimes you enjoy, like dance, yoga, or swimming.

• Get in contact with nature: Go outside and enjoy the sunshine and clean air. You can find inner peace and tranquility in nature, which is naturally serene.

• Prioritize your well-being and set boundaries: Saying no should not be feared. It's acceptable to decline pointless commitments when you need time to relax and recover.

Keep in mind that getting enough sleep and recovering from injuries are necessities rather than frills. Self-care is not a form of selfishness; it's an interest in your general prosperity, your connections, and your physical and psychological wellness. In this way, set out to focus on rest and recuperation in your life, and you'll see an energetic sparkle inside!

Bonus Advice: Share the bliss of sleep! Ask your loved ones to join you for relaxing pursuits like leisurely strolls in the evening or contemplative tea breaks. By cooperating, you could create a cascade of calm and wellbeing. There's going to be sunny mornings and sweet dreams! Make sleep a priority, and you'll witness your soul blossom with revitalized energy.

NOURISHING YOUR BODY FOR OPTIMAL ENERGY

Think of this: a source of vitality, a supply of food for the body and mind, and a body that is teeming with vibrant health. This is the beautiful gift of fuelling your body for optimal health, not some distant ideal.

Food affects everything from your emotions to your energy levels; it's not just fuel for your cells. So let's put less emphasis on diet drama and more on creating a meaningful, beautiful relationship with food that lets your soul shine!

1. Rekindle Your Energetic Side with Rainbow:

Think of fruits and vegetables as the powerful color wheel provided by nature. Every day, heap a kaleidoscope of colors onto your plate. Orange carrots are abundant in beta-carotene, red peppers are high in vitamin C, and leafy greens are high in iron.

2. Make Friends With Complex Carbs:

Despite the fact that they have an unfortunate standing, not all starches are made equivalent. Complex starches like yams, lentils, and entire grains can replace sweet cakes. These give supported energy, empowering your body and psyche to work ordinarily day in and day out.

3. Strength of Proteins:

Protein is the fundamental building block of life and is needed for energy production and muscle repair. Lean meats, fish, and eggs may provide you with energy and satisfaction, as can plant-based alternatives like lentils and tofu. Never forget that moderation is key, so don't overdo it!

4. The Hydration Hero:

The unsung energy hero is water. Physical and mental sluggishness result from dehydration.

Make it an objective to hydrate a day, and have a reusable container not far off as a suggestion to continue to taste.

5. Be Aware of Your Body:

Give up on meticulous meal planning! Observe the signals of hunger and fullness your body sends forth. Eat till you're satisfied, don't penalize yourself for indulging on rare occasions. It should make us happy to eat, not guilty.

6. Mindful Consumption:

Savor your food! Set away your phone, find a seat, and concentrate on the flavors, textures, and colors of your cuisine. Chew slowly and thoroughly, savoring each bite. You'll be surprised at how much happier you feel when you eat mindfully.

Recall that choosing conscious actions that revitalize your essence and allow you to live your greatest life is the key to fueling your body for optimal energy. Try new things, enjoy yourself, and let your radiant inner health radiate!

Bonus Advice: Use creativity! Cook wholesome meals with friends and family, explore nearby farmer's markets, and experiment with new recipes. Since food is meant to be shared, let your relationships be infused with the joy of providing nourishment for your body.

Now go forth and nourish your soul! If you can cultivate a little awareness and a positive outlook, you can access a stream of energy that drives every aspect of your life. Become the happiest, healthiest version of yourself, and feel your essence sparkle with more vitality!

CHAPTER 5: CONNECTING WITH PURPOSE

Within you is a hidden element, a hidden fuel for your essence - your mission. It is the spark that fires your passion, gives your life significance, and provides direction for your energies. It isn't always simple to find, but the voyage itself is an exciting experience!

1.Discovering Your Inner Compass:

•Consider broad questions such as, "What makes you tick?" What type of legacy do you wish to leave behind? What activities energize you from the inside out?

•Consider your interests: What activities cause you to lose track of time? What abilities do you possess naturally? What subjects excite you in conversation?

•Think about your values: What means a lot to you?What principles govern your decisions? What reasons elicit empathy and compassion in you?

•Look for ideas: Read biographies of people who inspire you, watch films about worthwhile causes, and volunteer in various places. Open your eyes and let the world inspire you!

2.Getting in Touch with Your Spark:

•Pay attention to your intuition: Often, your gut instinct is your inner compass whispering sweet nothings about your mission. Pay heed to its cues and don't be scared to take risks.

•Don't wait for absolute clarity: your mission may not be a flash of insight. It often happens step by step, through modest actions and relationships made along the road.

•Accept the journey: Discovering your purpose is a never-ending adventure, not a one-time destination. Detours and bottlenecks should not discourage you; instead, view them as learning opportunities and continue exploring.

•Put your values into action: Align your actions with your basic values. When you live truly, your purpose emerges organically in your everyday choices.

Remember that connecting with your mission isn't about being famous or changing the world on your own. It is about discovering something in your life that makes you feel truly fulfilled, driven, and connected to something more than yourself.

Allow your mission to guide you, fueling your essence with passion and significance. Every move you take, every moment you live with intention, adds a glimmer to your inner fire.

Bonus Tip: Share your mission! Talk to your friends and family about what motivates you, look for groups with similar beliefs, and work together on initiatives that light your collective spark. You can generate a ripple effect of purpose that energizes everyone around you if you work together.

Go forth and discover your spark! You'll uncover the magnificent purpose that nourishes your soul and adds dynamic vitality to every element of your life if you keep an open mind and an inquisitive heart.

REDISCOVERING YOUR PASSION

Life might feel like a dusty attic at times, with cobwebs of monotony, boxes of commitments, and your shining enthusiasm buried somewhere in the muck. But don't worry, explorer! It isn't simply imaginable to rediscover your energy; it is likewise the way to enliven your pith and fill your existence with fundamental energy.

Bring Out Your Inner Explorer:

•Dive into your memories: Remember what made your heart sing when you were a kid? Was it creating bright worlds, erecting huge castles, or becoming lost in stories? These early hobbies might provide insight into your primary interests.

•Shake things up! Break free from habits! Try a new class, discover a secret area of your city, or volunteer for a worthy cause. Getting out of your comfort zone might rekindle lost interests.

•Utilize your senses: feel the warmth of the sun on your skin, the flavor of a good meal, or the melody of a favorite song. Expanded mindfulness could prompt unforeseen wellsprings of motivation.

•Interact with others. Share your findings with friends, family, and mentors. Their viewpoints might sometimes help you see yourself and your hobbies in a fresh way.

Relight the Fire:

•Begin small: Don't try to change your entire life. Choose something simple, such as a monthly pottery class or joining a book club devoted to a genre you enjoy.

•Accept flaws: Don't be concerned about being "good" at anything new. The delight of the journey, not the pressure of the destination, is at the heart of rediscovering your passion.

•Playfully: Have fun! Approach your exploration with a feeling of wonder and levity. Remember that your passion should offer you joy, not worry.

Mark important anniversaries: Recognize your progress, no matter how minor. A triumph might be as simple as finishing a painting, writing a chapter, or simply turning up for your passion!

Keep in mind that passion isn't always a single, blazing blaze. It might be a mosaic of little interests, abilities, and beliefs that combine to provide a lively image of who you are.

Allow your rediscovered passion to be your guiding light, fueling your essence and illuminating your route to a life filled with joy and significance.

Bonus Tip: Spread the flame! Empower your loved ones to go with you on your journey of rediscovery. Investigate shared interests, empower each other, and celebrate each other's triumphs. You'll find that energy thrives locally among similar people.

So, explorer, set out! Your passion awaits rediscovery. You'll spark your soul and ignite a life that exudes brilliant energy if you have an inquisitive heart and an open mind. Remember, you are worth living a sparkling life!

ALIGNING YOUR ACTIVITIES WITH YOUR VALUES

Consider a compass within that guides your decisions toward a life that hums with joy and significance. That is the power of connecting your actions to your beliefs, the principles that hold your soul together. It's not about following certain rules, but rather about connecting into your inner knowledge and allowing it to illuminate the route to a more vibrant, invigorated self.

Finding Your Guiding Stars:

•Attend a values retreat: Consider what is most important to you. Is it generosity, ingenuity, ethics, or possibly adventure? Make a list of words that speak to you.

•Consider your options: What activities give you a sense of accomplishment? What decisions have you been conflicted about? Take note of how your values manifest in your daily life.

•Look for ideas: Read about individuals who live their ideals, watch films about communities founded on shared values, and learn from those who exude authenticity.

•Pose significant questions to yourself: When presented with a decision, ask yourself, "Does this align with my values?" When it comes to navigating the twists and turns of life, this straightforward inquiry can be a useful compass.

Living in Consonance with Your Compass:

•Small steps, great results: Begin by matching modest chores to your ideals. Choose a meal that shows your devotion to health, work on a passion project that sparks your creativity, or volunteer for a cause near and dear to your heart.

•Accept flaws: Don't be disheartened by mistakes. Aligning your life with your principles is a process rather than a destination. Learn from your mistakes and gradually steer yourself back to your North Star.

•Communicate your values as follows: Share your values with your friends and family. This transparency encourages support and creates an atmosphere in which you may all thrive genuinely.

Celebrate your alignment by recognizing your success! Take a minute to enjoy the peace you create inside yourself when you make a choice that is in line with your ideals.

Remember that aligning your actions with your principles does not imply conforming to a template. It's about embracing your distinctive flame and allowing your principles to illuminate the path to a life that feels real and vibrant.

Allow your principles to be your guiding light, shining a bright glow of inner harmony on every step you take. You'll discover a new source of energy, a feeling of purpose, and a way of living that just feels right.

Share your ideals by dancing! Encourage your friends and family to investigate their own beliefs and discover methods to live truthfully together. Create a community where you can celebrate and encourage one other's individual adventures. You may generate a ripple effect of colorful life that brightens up the planet by working together.

So, explorer, go out! Your values are waiting to take you on an unforgettable trip toward a life that energizes your soul and allows you to shine from inside. Remember, you are deserving of living an authentic life!

CHAPTER 6: SOCIAL ENERGIZERS

Social relationships are like sparkling synapses, enhancing our happiness, motivation, and overall well-being. However, social batteries can run low at times, leaving us feeling depleted and isolated. This is where the power of social energizers comes into play! These are easy, conscious strategies to awaken your soul and exude vivid energy, attracting others and producing a joyful ripple effect.

Connect with purpose:

•Move beyond casual talk and go deeper into conversations. Ask open-ended questions, tell true tales, and honestly listen to the responses. When you open your heart, you'll be astonished at the relationships you make.

•Let go of routine and embrace unpredictability! Plan a last-minute picnic, sign up for a dancing lesson with pals, or simply stroll around a new area with them. New experiences produce shared memories and laughter, which is the ultimate energy booster.

•Celebrate differences: Diversity is a treasure trove, not a challenge! Accept other points of view, cultures, and backgrounds. Open your minds, learn from one another, and revel in the diversity of human experience.

Develop a playful spirit:

•Let your inner child go wild: Remember the games you used to enjoy as a kid? Play board games, hold a charades night, or construct a blanket castle. Laughter and hilarity spread like wildfire, leaving everyone energized and connected.

•Get moving together: From fun walks to spontaneous dance parties, physical activity is a powerful tool for social connection. It releases endorphins, improves mood, and fosters shared experiences that strengthen connections.

•Volunteer as a group: Giving back as a group is a great energizer. Find a cause that everyone is passionate about, donate your time, and experience the satisfaction of making a difference together.

Remember that social energizers aren't about forcing conversations or filling up your social calendar. It's about connecting with individuals who bring out the best in you, sharing true joy, and radiating your vivid soul into the world.

Make yourself the energizer bunny! Plan events, introduce individuals, and create environments where others may connect and grow. Your excitement will be contagious, and you will be surrounded by a group that will reinvigorate your essence every day.

So, social butterfly, go forth! Accept the power of connection, share your radiant light, and watch as your social circle transforms into a radiant center of shared joy and energy. Remember that you were born to shine, and people are drawn to your light.

BUILDING SUPPORTIVE CONNECTIONS

Life's path is a lot more exciting when shared with a supporting crew. These aren't simply "faint-hearted allies"—they're the team promoters uninvolved, the shoulders to sob on, and the voices murmuring empowering words when your light is blurring. Building these connections isn't a contest; rather, it is a superb demonstration of feeding your spirit and bringing pleasure into your life.

Creating the Groundwork for Friendship

• Be open and vulnerable: allow others to connect with your actual self by sharing honest stories, worries, and hopes. It builds trust and creates the basis for a helpful relationship.

• Listen actively: Put your phone down, make eye contact, and fully absorb what they're saying. Show them you care about their views and feelings, and watch your bond grow stronger.

• Assist others: Be the buddy who shows up, not just with words but also with acts. Allow your actions to speak louder than your words, whether it's a modest gesture like getting coffee or a larger show of support during a difficult time.

Celebrate their triumphs by becoming their biggest fan! Celebrate their accomplishments, large and small, and express your pride in their path.

Growing a Garden of Friendship:

• Make time, even if it's difficult. Life is busy, so prioritize your supporting relationships. Plan frequent catch-ups, send thoughtful notes, and show them how much they mean to you.

•Accept disagreements: Life isn't all sunshine and rainbows! Healthy disputes are an essential component of every good connection. Learn to interact politely, to listen to diverse points of view, and to establish common ground despite differences.

•create loving boundaries: Respect your own needs and create healthy limits. Saying "no" is sometimes vital to safeguard your energies and guarantee your personal well-being.

•Forgive and move on: Nobody, not even our friends, is flawless. Learn to forgive little errors, talk honestly, and let go of grudges. Concentrate on developing a friendship based on mutual understanding and respect.

Remember that developing supportive relationships requires time and effort. It's about developing a friendship garden, nourishing each link with love and care. As these relationships bloom, they will energize your essence and enhance your life with lively delight, steadfast support, and a strong feeling of belonging.

Bonus Tip: Be the buddy you're looking for! Offer assistance, actively listen, and rejoice in the accomplishments of others. By exuding warmth and generosity, you attract more of the same, resulting in a chain reaction of supporting relationships that energizes everyone around you.

So, friend-maker, go forth! Open your heart, offer a helping hand, and plant a garden of supporting relationships to nurture your essence and illuminate your path with steadfast love and vivid energy. You deserve to thrive in a community that sees, values, and loves you for who you actually are.

SETTING BOUNDARIES FOR HEALTHY RELATIONSHIPS

Consider your energy to be a blazing flame. It warms and brightens when it is close, yet it burns when it is too close. Setting appropriate boundaries in your relationships is like setting a safe distance around a flame, preserving its essence while enhancing its warmth. Here's how to keep your relationships glowing with joy:

1. Understand Your Flame:

• Determine your needs: What saps your energy? What activities excite you? Knowing your priorities is essential for determining where limits are required.

• Respect your boundaries: Don't overextend yourself to satisfy others. Saying "no" to conserve your energy is not selfish; it is self-care.

2. Create the Spark Guard:

• Honest communication: express your boundaries clearly and gently. Instead of saying, "Quit being irritating," take a stab at saying,

"When you do X, I feel Y." "Could we at any point track down another way?"

• Action speaks louder than words: respect your own limits. Demonstrate that "no" means "no" and that "time for me" is non-negotiable.

3. Rekindle Your Fire:

• Stimulate your spirit: Set aside a few minutes for things that rejuvenate you, like perusing, working out, or investing energy in nature.A full flame indicates a more visible connection.

• Keep a healthy distance: Give your loved ones their own place to shine. Trust that true connection coexists with healthy independence.

Bonus Tip: Boundaries are bridges, not barriers! They create a comfortable environment for free conversation, allowing relationships to grow deeper and stronger.

Remember that setting limits isn't about driving people away; it's about fostering healthy, energetic connections that fuel your essence and everyone around you. Shine brightly!

CHAPTER 7: ENERGIZING WORK AND PRODUCTIVITY

Work should not deplete your spirit; rather, it should energize it! Here are some tips for turning your workplace into a source of energy and accomplishment:

1. Power Up Your Inner Engine:

•Begin Strong: Get up and move with a nutritious breakfast. An energized body nourishes a concentrated mind.

•Enjoy Nature: Take pauses in the sun or in green settings. Natural light and fresh air boost your energy levels dramatically.

•Nosh and Hydrate: Don't allow low blood sugar or dehydration sap your energy. Always have water and nutritious foods on hand.

2. Work smarter rather than harder:

•Control the To-Do List: Prioritize with zeal. Perform the most challenging tasks first, and then reward yourself with simpler ones.

• The Pomodoro Method: Partition work into 25-minute overflows with brief intervals in the middle between. Concentrate like a laser, then relax your mind and body.

•Quiet the Noise: Notifications, clutter, and multitasking are all productivity killers. To enhance your flow, create a distraction-free zone.

3. Instill Joy in Your Environment:

•Personalize your workspace: Fill it with items that inspire and encourage you. Plants, photographs, or a cherished saying may make a big difference.

•Move it or lose it: Avoid being stuck to your chair. Keep your body and psyche dynamic by standing up, extending, and moving to a most optimized plan of attack.

•Celebrate triumphs: Perceive your achievements, regardless of how enormous or little. A congratulatory gesture spurs you to continue onward.

Remember that work-life balance is essential. Outside of work, prioritize things that feed your spirit. A happy and relaxed you provides vigor to your duties.

So, let your work shine your soul rather than burn you out! Your workplace may become a catapult for productivity and joy with a little TLC. Energized, go forth and conquer!

BALANCING WORKLOAD AND PERSONAL TIME

Have you ever felt like a juggling clown, juggling emails and errands, dreams and deadlines? Don't be concerned; you're not alone! The good news is that you may abandon your frenzied juggling act and find the miracle of balance. Here's how to replenish your spirit with a healthy mix of work and play:

1. Understand Your Rhythm:

•Be aware of your body's energy peaks and valleys. Schedule challenging work during your most alert hours and leave time for lighter activities when your concentration wanes.

•Know your limitations: Don't be a productivity martyr. Recognize your natural time limitations and minimize fatigue by arranging guilt-free relaxation.

2. Control the To-Do Monster:

•Plan like a pro: Set ruthless priorities. To avoid feeling overwhelmed, use lists and strategies to arrange your task.

•Learn to say no: Not everything is worth your time and effort. Refuse jobs that do not accord with your priorities or sap your soul.

•Delegate and automate: Can it be done by someone else? To save up time and mental space, delegate or automate repetitive jobs.

3. Feed Your Playful Spirit:

•Make time for joy: Don't wait for "someday" to live. Schedule time in your calendar for things that offer you delight, whether they be artistic endeavors, workouts, or comforting reads.

•Disconnect to reconnect: Put the phone down, close the laptop, and take a step away from the screen. Immerse yourself in the present moment, whether it's through a thoughtful stroll or a genuine chat with family and friends.

•Move your body, move your mood: Exercise is about more than simply your physical wellness. It's an excellent mood enhancer and stress reducer. Choose an activity that you like, such as dancing or hiking, and let your body move your anxieties away.

Remember, it's alright to make changes! Because life is fluid, your optimal balance may vary from time to time. Be adaptable, pay attention to your requirements, and don't be afraid to change your schedule or priorities as necessary.

So put the juggling pins away and enjoy the lively symphony of work and pleasure. When you nurture both, you create a lovely rhythm that energizes your essence and allows you to reach your greatest potential. Shine brightly!

ENHANCING PRODUCTIVITY THROUGH ENERGY MANAGEMENT

Feeling like your to-do list is never-ending and your energy levels are depleted? Stop pushing yourself and rediscover the joy of powering your job with your energy, rather than the other way around! Here's how to become a productivity powerhouse:

1. Understand Your Energy Flow:

• Track your peaks and dips: Your energy ebbs and flows like the tide. Determine when you are laser-focused and when you require a recharge.

•Schedule strategically: Prioritize difficult chores during your peak hours and postpone lighter activities for times when your concentration wanes.

2. Set priorities based on your passion:

•Embrace the "no": not everything is worth your time and attention. Accept jobs that do not connect with your goals or sap your soul.

• Pay attention to high-impact tasks: Identify the 2-3 items that make the biggest difference and prioritize them relentlessly. Less is definitely more!

3. Power Up Your Inner Engine:

• Feed your body: Don't run on empty!Pick nutritious dinners and snacks to keep your cerebrum and body fueled day in and day out.

•Move your body: Practice isn't just really great for your wellbeing; it is likewise a characteristic energy supporter. A stroll, dance break, or fast workout routine will get your blood pumping and your mind invigorated.

•Hydrate for Focus: Do you have a thirst? Your mind is probably parched as well! For maximum clarity and vitality, have a reusable water bottle nearby and sip away.

4. Establish a Sanctuary:

•Control the chaos: Clutter causes mental tiredness. Organize your workstation and eliminate distractions so you can focus with pinpoint accuracy.

•Embrace nature's power: Take pauses in natural light or green settings. Fresh air and sunshine boost your energy and attitude.

•Reduce the background noise: Notifications, multitasking, and continual bustle are productivity killers. To optimize your flow state, create a distraction-free zone.

5. Don't Forget About Having Fun:

•Plan joy breaks: Recharge your spirit with brief bursts of things you enjoy, such as reading a chapter, playing a small game, or talking with a friend.

• Celebrate triumphs: Each achievement, regardless of how extraordinary or little, should be perceived. Reward yourself and feed your motivation to keep going.

Bonus Tip: Pay attention to your intuition! Don't push yourself if you're exhausted. Take a pause, refresh, and return with renewed vigor.

Remember that a rested and revitalized you is a productive you!

So, let go of the burnout and discover your endless energy source within. By managing your energy, you can finish your plan for the day, yet you will likewise encounter the delight and satisfaction that come from working in a state of harmony with your regular stream. Go forward, fired up, and unstoppable!

CHAPTER 8: CREATIVITY AND PLAY

Our inner flame might flicker in the midst of regular existence, and our spirits can seem muted. However, buried under the regularity is a powerful force: a thriving playground of imagination and play. Let us revive the latent kid inside, rekindle our soul, and revitalize our lives with a playful twist today!

1. Use Your Senses to Paint: Ditch the brushes and canvases. Shut your eyes and imagine colors ejecting on your tongue as you eat up a succulent orange. Take in the cool morning air and let the daylight warm your skin. Exploration with your senses should be fun. Allow the world to be your canvas, and each experience to be a bright brush.

2. Dance As If No One Is Watching (Except Your Pet): Turn up the music, let go of inhibitions, and allow your body to become a conduit for delight. Own your rhythm by wriggling, twirling, stomping, and leaping. What does it matter if you're a ballerina or a breakdancer? It's your personal disco, your playground for unadulterated expression.

3. Create Cardboard Castles and Paper Dragons: Remember when construction paper and cardboard boxes were magical? Rekindle your sense of curiosity! Build a fantasy fort, create a fleet of origami boats, or bring a crumpled napkin dragon to life. Accept the innocent delight of creating, the rush of watching an idea come to life. There are no rules or expectations; just pure, fun imagination.

4. Play Games with an Adult Twist: Remember games like tag, hide-and-seek, or charades? Dust them off, but with an adult twist! Make charades into a Shakespearean play, make up ridiculous tag rules, or conceal clues for a treasure hunt that leads to a surprise picnic. Reimagine childhood games with a splash of wit and a dash of your own personality.

5.Laugh Until Your Sides Hurt: Find the ludicrous in the serious, and the comic in the commonplace. Watch a slapstick comedy, tell stupid jokes to your buddies, or simply enjoy the pleasure of a good belly laugh. Laughter is a powerful energy enhancer, a spark that lights the spirit on fire. Allow it to flow over you, removing cobwebs and leaving your soul light and lively.

Remember that creativity and play are not frills, but necessary components of a fulfilling existence. They reignite our fire, revitalize our essence, and remind us that life is, at its heart, a playground just waiting to be discovered. So go forth and paint with your senses, dance like a fool, create fantastical worlds, and let laughter lead you. Unleash your playful flame and see your soul come to life!

TAPPING INTO CREATIVE ENERGIES

We all have a creative wellspring within us, boiling just beneath the surface of our daily lives. However, the hurry of life can leave us feeling tired and distant from that lively spark. Let's go deep today and reconnect with our creative energy, reigniting our souls and infusing life with new possibilities!

1. Light a Match to Dry Leaves Curiosity: Remember when you were a kid and every leaf contained a mystery and every puddle was a portal? Rekindle your interest! Ask "why?" about everything, venture down new roads, and revel in the thrill of discovery. Watch a video on an unusual species, go to a free poetry reading, or simply walk through a new neighborhood—allow your curiosity to be the compass that leads you to inspiration.

2. Shake Up Your Routine, Spice Up Your Spice Rack: The familiar might put us to sleep creatively. Break the cycle! Take an alternative route to work, prepare food from a different cuisine, or enroll in a new workout class. Experiment with stepping outside your comfort zone in minor ways to notice how it opens your mind and stimulates new thoughts.

3. Daydream Like a Cloud Gazer: We frequently overlook the potential of pure daydreaming in our fast-paced environment. Allow yourself time to simply let your mind roam. Create sky castles, individuals with bizarre idiosyncrasies, or vividly design your ideal trip. Allow your thoughts to wander freely, without judgment or restraint, and see where the creative wind leads you.

4. Use a Butterfly Net to Capture Inspiration: Don't let ephemeral thoughts flutter away! Keep a scratch pad, make voice accounts on your telephone, or even doodle primer diagrams on napkins. Catch those glimmerings of motivation before they disappear, and support them into undeniable imaginative thoughts.

5. Make Friends with Other Explorers: Creativity flourishes in the community. Take part in a canvas class, a composing club, or a web-based craftsmanship gathering. Encircle yourself with other people who share your advantage so you might run thoughts by each other and gain from their encounters.

Keep in mind that creative energy is not a finite resource but rather a wellspring that grows with use. The more you tap into it, the greater the flow. So go forth, pique your interest, mix up your routine, fantasize freely, collect ideas, and connect with your creative community. Unleash the lively flow within you and witness your essence come to life with the power of creativity!

EMBRACING PLAY AND LEISURE

We frequently overlook the key flame that feeds our greatest delight in our tireless quest of productivity: recreation and leisure. These are not frivolous pleasures, but powerful weapons for replenishing our spirits, reigniting our passions, and instilling life with a lively sense of wonder. Today, let's get off the hamster wheel, reclaim our inner playground, and re-energize our soul via the power of play!

1. Rediscover the Joy of "Just Because": Remember when you were a kid and you used to create forts out of blankets and pillows because it felt like pure magic? Rekindle that carefree spirit! Make pancakes simply for the sake of flipping them, dance to your favorite music even if no one is looking, or color outside the lines for the sake of it. Accept the thrill of doing things just for the sake of doing them, with no aim or objective in mind.

2. Make Errands Into Adventures: Let's face it, going food shopping may be a hassle. But what if it was a hunt for the most delicious ingredients? Or what about a culinary scavenger hunt? Incorporate fun twists into your regular routine. Make a stroll become a nature walk, a commute into a sing-along, or cleaning into a dance party. The options are limitless!

3. Be a "Yes" Person to Spontaneous Fun: Say "yes" to unexpected activities instead of tight timetables! Join friends for a last-minute picnic, ride your bike around a new area, or just say "yes" to that ridiculous game your inner kid is pushing you to do. Accept the unexpected, the unplanned, and the deliciously silly moments that bring you joy and laughter.

4. Reconnect with Your Inner Child: Remember when there was no limit to your playing and your creativity reigned supreme?

Reconnect with your fun side! Read a favorite childhood novel, make a sandcastle on the beach, or host a tea party with plush animals. Allow your inner child to guide you, rediscover simple pleasures, and watch your soul come alive with youthful wonder.

5. Make Time for "Nothingness": In our never-ending pursuit of busyness, we frequently overlook the potential of just being. Schedule unstructured time in your day to just "be." Read a book without looking at your phone, go on a stroll without a plan, or simply relax and watch the clouds pass by. Allow yourself the gift of peaceful thought, and allow the enchantment of "nothingness" to rejuvenate your spirit.

Remember that play and leisure are acts of self-care that nourish our souls and invigorate our own essence, not symptoms of weakness. So go off and construct forts, chase butterflies, sing like no one is listening, and revel in the enchantment of the unexpected. Allow your inner child to lead the way, and watch your life come alive with the colorful energy of play!

CHAPTER 9: OVERCOMING OBSTACLES

Life is like a mountain route, meandering and lovely yet strewn with stones and vegetation. These hurdles, no matter how great or minor, may leave us exhausted and disheartened. But keep in mind that real essence lives on struggle! Let us learn today to cross the tough spots, turn barriers into stepping stones, and emerge even stronger with a bright, energetic spirit!

1. Change Your Perspective: From Roadblock to Stepping Stone: Every adversity contains a hidden lesson, an opportunity to learn and grow. View it as a diversion to a new peak rather than a dead end. "What can I learn from this?" ask yourself. "How can it help me grow stronger?" This adjustment in viewpoint will strengthen your resolve and transform dissatisfaction into fuel for progress.

2. Break it down into steps: Overwhelmed by a massive boulder? Don't attempt to push it all the way upward! Divide it into smaller, more manageable parts. Put forth momentary objectives, praise every smaller than usual triumph, and you'll end up crawling nearer to the top. Recollect that even the most considerable mountains should be scaled mindfully.

3. Seek Help, Not Shortcuts: We are not designed to climb alone. Make contact with your tribe! Speak with your friends, family, mentors, or even online groups. Share your difficulties, get guidance, and draw strength from their common experiences. Remember that a helping hand may make even the most difficult slopes less intimidating.

4. Appreciate the Detours: The road to the top is rarely straight up. Accept the unforeseen diversions! Perhaps you take a wrong turn and come into a secret waterfall, or perhaps a thunderstorm drives you to seek shelter, bringing you to a nice café serving the greatest hot chocolate in town. Remember that even detours may be magical in their own right, bringing unexpected beauty and richness to your journey.

5. Find Fuel in Your Passion: What makes your heart sing? What lights your spirit on fire? When faced with a challenge, remember your passion. Permit it to act as your compass and directing light, helping you to remember why you're rising this mountain in any case. With enthusiasm as your fuel, you'll have the energy to conquer any obstruction.

Remember that problems are not hurdles, but rather chances to climb above and unleash your inner strength. Accept the struggle, learn from the diversions, and never lose sight of the spectacular vista that awaits you at the top. When you do, your essence will be rejuvenated, your spirit will soar, and you will be able to climb any mountain life throws your way!

IDENTIFYING AND OVERCOMING BARRIERS TO RECOVERY

Recovery is a process rather than a destination. And, like with any voyage, there will be stunning vistas and unforeseen detours. However, such diversions might sometimes feel more like hurdles, obstacles that threaten to dull our healing flame. Let us shine light on finding these hurdles and using the strength inside to burst past them, reigniting our essence and invigorating our journey to well-being today!

Bringing the Shadows to Light:

Recognizing the presence of any barrier is the first step toward conquering it. Here are some common stumbling blocks you may face on your way to recovery:

Negative self-talk: Your inner critic may be a tyrant, spewing doubt and negativity. Remember, it's not your truth; it's simply a voice you may choose to ignore.

Fear of relapse: Relapse is an inevitable aspect of many recovery journeys and is not a failure. Learn from it, get back up, and keep going ahead.

Isolation and loneliness: Seeking help is critical. Connect with loved ones, support groups, or therapists if you feel alone.

Identify your triggers and build healthy coping techniques to help you navigate them without being carried away.

Loss of motivation: It's normal to feel disheartened from time to time. Celebrate your minor victories, seek inspiration, and recall why you began this path in the first place.

Breakthrough Tools for Empowerment:

Let's equip ourselves with instruments to illuminate the route ahead now that we've discovered the shadows:

Self-compassion is being kind with oneself. Setbacks should be viewed as learning opportunities rather than personal failures.

Pay attention to your thoughts and feelings with mindfulness and self-awareness. This awareness allows you to make intentional decisions rather than being swept away by emotions.

Develop healthy coping techniques, such as exercise, journaling, or spending time in nature, to reduce stress and cravings.

Surround yourself with individuals who care about and support your rehabilitation. Don't be hesitant to ask for assistance.

Celebration and self-care: Celebrate your tiny and large successes. Make self-care activities that feed your mind, body, and soul a priority. Keep in mind that rehabilitation is a marathon, not a sprint.

Remember that you are in good company this way. You have the inner power and resilience to face any challenge. Accept the obstacles, appreciate your accomplishments, and most importantly, never lose sight of the vivid, powerful soul that is inside you!

Allow the beauty of the sunrise to serve as a reminder that even the darkest night gives way to a fresh morning. Believe in your ability to overcome obstacles, re energize your essence, and recover your well-being. You can do it!

LEARNING FROM SETBACKS

Life is a lovely adventure, but it is rarely easy. We all have setbacks, missteps, and instances when things do not go as planned. These encounters may be disheartening, leaving us drained and questioning our progress. However, it is during difficult times that we have the opportunity to learn, grow, and re-energize our own essence.

Recognizing setbacks as stepping stones

Shifting our viewpoint is the key to turning failures into stepping stones. We might regard them as opportunities for learning and progress rather than as impediments. We may learn useful lessons from even the most difficult circumstances if we ask the correct questions and adopt a development attitude.

When faced with a setback, consider the following questions:

What can I take away from this encounter?

What might I have done better?

What can I do to grow stronger and more resilient as a result of this?

What simple measures can I take to progress?

Remember that setbacks do not define us; rather, they polish us. Each obstacle we conquer molds us into better, wiser versions of ourselves.

Using Growth to Your Advantage

It's time to put the lessons we've learned from our setbacks into action now that we've identified them. Here are some strategies for harnessing the power of development and re-energizing your essence:

Celebrate your modest victories: Every small step forward is a victory. Recognize your progress and appreciate your tenacity.

Embrace continual learning: Never stop learning and broadening your views. Read books, attend classes, and surround yourself with people who inspire you.

Self-compassion: Be compassionate to oneself, especially during difficult circumstances. Forgive yourself and concentrate on going forward.

Discover your source of inspiration: What drives you? What piques your interest? Reconnect with your mission and allow it to lead you through difficult times.

Remember that while setbacks are transient, the lessons we acquire from them are eternal. We may invigorate our essence and emerge from every mishap stronger and more vibrant than before by adopting a growth mentality and viewing obstacles as chances to learn and improve.

So, the next time you face a setback, take a deep breath, change your viewpoint, and consider it as an opportunity to shine. The lessons you acquire will not only assist you in overcoming this obstacle, but will also prepare you for the thrilling experiences that await you.

Believe in yourself and your potential to learn, grow, and prosper. Your essence is ready to be charged!

CONCLUSION

As we close the book on "Energize Your Essence: A Comprehensive Recovery Blueprint," take a minute to reflect on the transforming trip you've been on. This last chapter acts as a compass, taking you through the important parts of reflection and the road map for living an invigorated life.

Your Recovery Journey in Review

Accepting Progress

Recognize your accomplishments in understanding and regaining your energy.

Celebrate the minor successes and acknowledge the good improvements that have occurred during your recovery path.

Learning from Difficulties

Consider the difficulties encountered and the lessons learnt. Every adversity is a chance for progress. Consider how these difficulties have formed your resilience and inspired your passion to live a rich life.

Developing Self-Compassion

As you reflect on your trip, be kind to yourself. Recognize that rehabilitation is a journey, and that each step you take demonstrates your commitment to a better, more energetic life.

Maintaining an Energized Lifestyle

Practice Integration

Investigate methods to incorporate the practices and strategies taught in this blueprint into your everyday routine. Small, focused actions multiplied over time provide a foundation for long-term vitality.

Taking Care of Your Essence

Make a continuous commitment to self-care and nourishment. Recognize that maintaining enthusiastic living necessitates constant attention to your physical, emotional, and mental well-being. Set aside time for activities that will refill your energy reserves.

Increasing Resilience

Accept challenges with renewed vigor. Develop a mindset that sees failures as chances for re-calibration, strengthening your capacity to negotiate life's ebbs and flows with grace and drive.

Finally, "Energize Your Essence" is more than just a guide; it is a companion on your continual path toward a life full of energy and meaning. May the insights acquired and techniques adopted help you to survive and preserve the invigorated life you've nurtured along this inspiring journey.

www.ingramcontent.com/pod-product-compliance
Lightning Source LLC
Chambersburg PA
CBHW070946260726
48661CB00003B/1152